RHINOPLASTY: WHAT EVERY PATIENT NEEDS TO KNOW

BRENTON B. KOCH M.D.

TRUST YOUR NOSE TO AN EXPERT WHO KNOWS!

Essential Considerations for Cosmetic Surgery Rhinoplasty Edition

Trust Your Nose To An Expert Who Knows!

Essential Considerations for Cosmetic Surgery

Rhinoplasty Edition

Copyright © 2012 Brenton B. Koch M.D.

All rights reserved.

ISBN: 1479344818

ISBN 13: 9781479344819

The information contained in this book is intended to provide helpful and informative material on the subject addressed. It is not intended to serve as a replacement for professional medical advice. Any use of the information in this book is at the reader's discretion. The author and publisher specifically disclaim any and all liability arising directly or indirectly from the use or application of any information contained in this book. A health care professional should be consulted regarding your specific situation. Bottom line; ask your doctor.

PROCEDURE: COSMETIC RHINOPLASTY

(Surgery to improve the appearance of my nose.)

Table of Contents

- About The Author — v
- Introduction — vii
- Surgery Of The Nose — 1
- Is Rhinoplasty For You? — 3
- Making The Decision For Rhinoplasty — 5
- Understanding The Surgery — 7
- Preparing For Surgery General — 9
- Two Weeks Before Surgery — 11
- The Day Before Surgery — 13
- The Morning Of Surgery — 15
- Medications To Avoid Before And After Surgery — 17
- Ibuprofen Medications to Avoid — 21
- Other Medications to Avoid — 23
- Tricyclic Antidepressant Medications to Avoid — 25
- Going To The Surgery Center — 27
- The Recovery Area — 29
- General Surgical Risks — 31
- Normal Symptoms — 33
- Risks — 35
- Rarer Complications — 37
- Unsatisfactory Result & Need For Revisional Surgery — 39
- Specific Surgical Risks Rhinoplasty (Nose Reshaping) — 41
- Applicable Health Factors — 43

- Other Risks And Information 45
- Medications 49
- Instructions 51
- Postoperative Care Outpatient Surgery Your First 48 Hours 53
- Specific Post Operative Instructions Rhinoplasty (Nose Reshaping) 55
- As You Heal 57
- Specific As You Heal Information Rhinoplasty (Nose Reshaping) 59
- Longer Term Postoperative Instructions 61
- Finally 63

About the Author

Brenton Koch, MD, FACS, is a board-certified facial plastic and reconstructive surgeon. He is certified by both the American Board of Facial Plastic and Reconstructive Surgery and the American Board of Otolaryngology - Head and Neck Surgery. At his practice in Des Moines, Iowa, plastic surgery of the face is his exclusive specialty. Dr. Koch is supported by administrative and operating room staffs that are specifically trained to care for plastic and reconstructive surgery patients. Each year this team of professionals prepares for and performs hundreds of facial surgeries treating conditions relating to appearance, accident, or disease.

Dr. Koch completed his undergraduate and pre-medical training at Drake University in Des Moines. He graduated from the University of Iowa College of Medicine, where he received numerous honors including the Hancher-Finkbine Medallion for outstanding academic leadership contributions to the University of Iowa College of Medicine. He also earned the American Medical Association National Leadership Achievement Award, which is presented to only twenty recipients nationally.

Dr. Koch completed residency at the prestigious University of Iowa Department of Otolaryngology - Head and Neck Surgery, which consistently ranks as one of the top programs in the country. He subsequently completed advanced fellowship training in facial plastic and reconstructive surgery at Indiana University and the Meridian Plastic Surgery Center in Indianapolis through the American Academy of Facial Plastic and Reconstructive Surgery. He served as clinical instructor of facial plastic surgery at Indiana University, and is currently a clinical instructor of facial plastic surgery with the University of Iowa Department of Otolaryngology - Head and Neck Surgery. He has continued to maintain active involvement in clinical research, with numerous publications, research awards and national presentations to his credit.

Dr. Koch and his wife, Heidi M. Koch MD, an age management and functional medicine physician, reside in Des Moines with their four children: Nicole, Blake, Tatum and Piper. Dr. Koch enjoys sports of all kinds, and as a former college football player, Ironman and competitive bodybuilder, he avidly enjoys exercise. His favorite activities, however, are those spent with his family.

Dr. Koch is the founder of a charitable non-profit for underprivileged student athletes called Empower to Play, an avid supporter of numerous charitable organizations in his community such as the Animal Rescue League of Iowa, Juvenile Diabetes Research Foundation, Mercy Medical Center's Mammogram Assistance Fund and countless others through donations of his time and services.

Introduction

Congratulations! Your purchase of this book is the first step in having a confident and clear understanding of the cosmetic surgery you may be considering.

The questions, expectations and recommendations contained in this book will be vital to your outcome. This book will give insight into the realities of cosmetic surgery, reasons you may or may not choose to have surgery at all and secrets for a successful recovery.

The decision to have cosmetic surgery is a serious one and should not be made hastily. Review this book a number of times. Highlight sections or "dog-ear" pages and take this along to your consultation so you can remember all the questions you want to ask your surgeon. Remember, the more information you have, the more prepared both you and your surgeon will be prior to surgery.

As a cosmetic surgeon, I recommend you get a number of opinions regarding your options. Go to at least 2 or 3 consultations and ASK QUESTIONS! It is common that I meet with my patients a number of times prior to surgery to make sure they have all of their questions answered before deciding to schedule surgery. Your surgeon should be willing to spend time with you personally and be open-minded to your questions. If at any time you feel pressured, put off, or feel you are getting the "hard sell," seek another opinion!

Cosmetic surgery is not free, but please, do not "bargain-shop" with your well-being. As the old saying goes, if it sounds too good to be true, it probably is. This is never more applicable than in cosmetic surgery.

It is with my best wishes for success and happiness with your cosmetic surgery outcome that I thank you for your purchase of this edition of Essential Considerations for Cosmetic Surgery.

Brenton B. Koch, M.D., F.A.C.S.
www.kochmd.com

Surgery of The Nose

Every year, half a million people who are interested in improving the appearance of their noses seek consultation with facial plastic surgeons. Some are unhappy with the noses they were born with, and some with the way aging has changed their nose. For others, an injury may have distorted the nose, or the goal may be improved breathing. But one fact is clear: Nothing has a greater impact on how a person looks than the size and shape of the nose. Because the nose is the most defining characteristic of the face, even a slight alteration can greatly improve one's appearance.

If you have wondered how nose surgery, or rhinoplasty, could improve your looks, self-confidence, or health, you need to know how rhinoplasty is performed and what you can expect. No book can allay all your concerns, but this one can provide answers for many of the questions you may have.

Successful facial plastic surgery is a result of good rapport between patient and surgeon. Trust, based on realistic expectations and exacting medical expertise, develops in the consulting stages before surgery. Your surgeon can answer, and should be willing to, specific questions about your unique needs.

Is Rhinoplasty For You?

As with all facial plastic surgery, good health and realistic expectations are prerequisites. Understanding nasal surgery is also critical. Since there is no ideal in rhinoplasty, the goal is to improve the nose aesthetically, making it harmonize better with other facial features.

Skin type, ethnic background, and age are important factors to be considered in discussions with your surgeon prior to surgery. Before the nose is altered, a young patient must reach full growth, usually around age fifteen or sixteen. Exceptions are cases in which breathing is severely impaired.

Before deciding on rhinoplasty, ask your surgeon if any additional surgery might be recommended to enhance the appearance of your face. For example, many patients have chin augmentation in conjunction with rhinoplasty to create a better balance of features.

Making The Decision For Rhinoplasty

Whether the surgery is desired for functional or cosmetic reasons, your choice of a qualified facial plastic surgeon is of paramount importance. Many facial plastic surgeons are trained in both ear, nose, throat, and facial cosmetic surgery, which provides you, the patient, with the highest level of training and expertise. Your surgeon will examine the structure of your nose, both externally and internally, to evaluate what you can expect from rhinoplasty. You are most likely to be pleased with the results of your surgery if you have a realistic idea of what nasal surgery can and cannot do.

You should expect a thorough explanation of your surgeon's expectations and the risks involved in surgery. Following a joint decision by you and your surgeon to proceed with rhinoplasty consultation, he or she will take photographs of you and discuss the options available. Your surgeon will explain how the nasal structures, including bone and cartilage, can be sculpted to reshape the nose and may indicate how reshaping the chin, for example, could enhance the desired results.

After conducting a thorough medical history, your surgeon will offer information regarding anesthesia, the surgical facility to be used, and the costs for the procedure. These costs may be combined in one fee or may be separated. Anesthesiologists or nurse anesthetists, for example, may be completely independent of your surgeon and therefore have a separate fee structure. The facility where you have surgery may be within your surgeon's practice or an independent center.

Understanding The Surgery

The definition of rhinoplasty is, literally, reshaping the nose. The etymology of the English word of rhinoplasty is derived from the Greek prefix "rhino" meaning nose, and "plasty" defined as a surgical procedure for the repair or restoration of a body part.

First, incisions are made and the bone and cartilage support system of the nose is accessed. The majority of incisions are made inside the nose, where they are invisible. In some cases, an incision is made in the area of skin separating the nostrils. Ask your surgeon about what incisions may be necessary. Next, certain amounts of underlying bone and cartilage are removed, added to, or rearranged to provide a newly shaped structure. For example, when the tip of the nose is too large, your surgeon may sculpt the cartilage in this area to reduce it in size. The angle of the nose and its relationship to the upper lip can be altered for a more youthful look or to correct an unusual difference.

The skin and overlying tissues are then re-draped over the newly reshaped frame and the incisions are closed. A splint is applied to the outside of the nose to help form and retain the new shape while the nose heals. Soft, absorbent material may or may not be used inside the nose to maintain stability along the dividing wall of the air passages, called the septum. Alternatively, soft nasal supports that permit nasal breathing post-operatively can be placed. Fortunately, the days of "packing the nose" are behind us and many surgeons place nothing at all in the nose after surgery.

Preparing For Surgery General

PRE-OP VISIT: You will likely have a pre-operative visit with your surgeon within several weeks prior to your surgery date. At this visit, he/she will review your medical history and complete a physical examination. He/She will discuss the procedure again within you and you are encouraged to ask questions you may still have. Depending on your general health, you may be asked to have an evaluation by your primary care medical provider to assure you are safe to proceed with surgery.

POSTOPERATIVE WOUND CARE SUPPLIES: At your pre-op visit, you may be provided with a kit of wound care supplies that will suffice for the entire recovery in most situations. If not, essential supplies include: saline nasal spray, cotton-tipped swabs, Vaseline, skin safe tape, 2x2 sponges/gauzes and the phone number to call your surgeon in case of questions or concerns that may arise after surgery.

LINE UP YOUR SUPPORT SYSTEM: You will need a family member or friend to drive you home from surgery and stay with you the first night because you will be somewhat sedated from the medications used during surgery.

HOUSEHOLD PREPARATION: Prepare and/or freeze several meals. This will allow you to take it easy for a few days, but still get a good diet that will promote rapid healing. Stock up on foods that won't require much chewing, such as yogurt, pudding, soup and applesauce. You might find it more convenient to purchase these in individual containers. It may be suggested you rest with your head elevated above your heart after surgery to help reduce swelling postoperatively. Determine where you will sleep whether it will be in a recliner, comfortable couch or propped-up by 3-4 pillows in bed.

Two Weeks Before Surgery

STOP SMOKING: Smoking reduces circulation to the skin and impedes healing. Smoking must be discontinued two weeks before surgery and two weeks after surgery, but longer is preferable.

TAKE MULTIVITAMINS: Start taking multivitamins daily to improve your general health once you have scheduled your surgery. Choose a multivitamin with less than 400 mg in Vitamin E. High doses of Vitamin E can lead to more bruising and bleeding at the time of surgery.

TAKE VITAMIN C: Start taking 500 mg of Vitamin C daily to promote healing.

DO NOT TAKE ASPIRIN OR IBUPROFEN FOR TWO WEEKS BEFORE AND TWO WEEKS AFTER SURGERY: Stop taking medications containing aspirin or ibuprofen. Review the list of drugs containing aspirin and ibuprofen carefully. Such drugs can cause bleeding problems during and after surgery. Instead, use medications containing acetaminophen (such as Tylenol).

DO NOT TAKE HERBAL MEDICATIONS: Many herbs can interact with anesthesia, cause bleeding or fluctuation of the blood pressure. For example, gingko biloba can reduce platelets, which are blood cells that are essential for clotting; ginseng can cause high blood pressure; and St. John's Wort may prolong the effects of anesthetic drugs.

LIMIT VITAMIN E: Limit your intake of Vitamin E to less than 400 mg per day.

FILL YOUR PRESCRIPTIONS: You will be likely be given prescriptions for medications. Please have them filled BEFORE the day of surgery.

ILLNESS: If you develop a cold, fever blisters, facial sores, or any other illness prior to surgery, please notify your doctor.

The Day Before Surgery

CONFIRM SURGERY TIME: The day before your procedure, you will likely be called to confirm the time of your surgery. If you are not going to be at home or at your office, please call the-office or surgery center to confirm the time of arrival and the time of your surgery.

CLEANSING: The night before surgery, shower and wash the surgical areas thoroughly with soap.

EATING AND DRINKING: Do not eat or drink anything after 12:00 midnight. This includes water. You may brush your teeth.

The Morning Of Surgery

SPECIAL INFORMATION: Do not eat or drink anything! If you take a daily medication, you may take it with a sip of water in the early morning. Ask your surgeon about this prior to surgery.

ORAL HYGIENE: You may brush your teeth, but do not swallow the water.

CLEANSING: Shower and wash the surgical areas again with soap.

MAKE-UP: Please do not wear moisturizers, creams, lotions, makeup, hairspray, or hair styling products.

CLOTHING: Wear only comfortable, loose fitting clothing that do not go over your head. Do not wear hairpins, hairpieces, and jewelry. Please do not bring valuables with you.

SOCKS: Bring warm socks to use during and after surgery.

CHECK-IN/PREPARATION: Confirm your surgery time. Report to the surgery center early. You should plan to arrive 60 minutes earlier than your scheduled surgery time. Patients less than 18 years old must be accompanied by a parent or legal guardian because legal consent forms will be reviewed. If the surgery center is separate from your physician's office, you will likely be asked to fill out additional paperwork when you check in. It's a good idea to check with the surgery center prior to surgery to determine what paperwork may be needed or if any payment may be necessary at the time of check in.

Medications To Avoid Before And After Surgery

If you are taking any medications on this list, they should be discontinued two weeks prior to surgery and only acetaminophen (i.e., Tylenol) should be taken for pain. Your doctor prior to surgery must specifically clear all other medications that you are currently taking. These lists are recommendations only and may be used as a guideline. They are not all inclusive lists. It is absolutely necessary that your doctor and the nursing staff prior to surgery specifically clear all of your current medications. These medications may be resumed two weeks following surgery. If you have questions about your medications, ask!

Aspirin Medications to Avoid

4-Way Cold Tabs
5-Aminosalicylic Acid
Acetylsalicylic Acid
Adprin-B products
Alka-Seltzer products
Amigesic
Anacin products
Anexsia w/Codeine
Argesic-SA
Arthra-G
Arthriten products
Arthritis Foundation products
Arthritis Pain formula
Arthritis Strength BC Powder
Arthropan
ASA

Asacol
Ascriptin products
Aspergum
Asprimox products
Axotal
Azdone
Azulfidine products
B-A-C
Backache Maximum Strength Relief
Bayer Products
BC Powder
Bismatrol products
Buffered Aspirin
Bufferin products
Buffetts 11
Buffex
Butal/ASA/Caff
Butalbital Compound
Cama Arthritis Pain Reliever
Carisoprodol Compound
Cheracol
Choline Magnesium Trisalicylate
Choline Salicylate
Cope
Coricidin
Cortisone Medications
Damason-P
Darvon Compound – 65
Darvon/ASA
Dipentum
Disalcid
Doan's products
Dolobid
Dristan
Duragesic
Easprin
Ecotrin products

Empirin products
Equagesic
Excedrin products
Fiorgen PF
Fiorinal products
Gelpirin
Genprin
Gensan
Goody's Extra Strength Headache Powders
Halfprin products
Isollyl Improved
Kaodene
Lanorinal
Lortab ASA
Magan
Magnaprin products
Magnesium Salicylate
Magsal
Marnal
Marthritic
Meprobamate
Mesalamine
Methocarbamol
Micrainin
Mobidin
Mobigesic
Momentum
Mono-Gesic
Night-Time Effervescent Cold
Norgesic products
Norwich products
Olsalazine
Orphengesic products
Oxycodone
Pabalate products
P-A-C
Pain Reliever Tabs

Panasal
Pentasa
Pepto-Bismol
Percodan products
Phenaphen/Codeine #3
Pink Bismuth
Propoxyphene Compound products
Robaxisal
Rowasa
Roxiprin
Saleto products
Salflex
Salicylate products
Salsalate
Salsitab
Scot-Tussin Original 5-Action
Sine-off
Sinutab
Sodium Salicylate
Sodol Compound
Soma Compound
St. Joseph Aspirin
Sulfasalazine
Supac
Suprax
Synalgos-DC
Talwin
Triaminicin
Tricosal
Trilisate
Tussanil DH
Tussirex products
Ursinus-Inlay
Vanquish
Wesprin
Willow Bark products
Zorprin

Ibuprofen Medications to Avoid

Actron
Acular (ophthalmic)
Advil products
Aleve
Anaprox products
Ansaid
Cataflam
Clinoril
Daypro
Diclofenac
Dimetapp Sinus
Dristan Sinus
Etodolac
Feldene
Fenoprofen
Flurbiprofen
Genpril
Haltran
IBU
Ibuprin
Ibuprofen
Ibuprohm
Indochron E-R
Indocin products
Indomethacin products
Ketoprofen
Ketorolac
Lodine
Meclofenamate

Meclomen
Mefenamic Acid
Menadol
Midol products
Motrin products
Nabumetone
Nalfon products
Naprelan
Naprosyn products
Naprox X
Naproxen
Nuprin
Ocufen (ophthalmic)
Orudis products
Oruvail
Oxaprozin
Piroxicam
Ponstel
Profenal
Relafen
Rhinocaps
Sine-Aid products
Sulindac
Suprofen
Tolectin products
Tolmetin
Toradol
Voltaren

Other Medications to Avoid

4-Way w/ Codeine
A.C.A.
A-A Compound
Acutrim
Actifed
Anexsia
Anisindione
Anturane
Arthritis Bufferin
BC Tablets
Children's Advil
Clinoril C
Contac
Coumadin
Dalteparin injection
Dicumarol
Dipyridamole
Doxycycline
Emagrin
Enoxaparin injection
Flagyl
Fragmin injection
Furadantin
Garlic
Heparin
Hydrocortisone
Isollyl
Lovenox injection
Macrodantin

Mellaril
Miradon
Opasal
Pan-PAC
Pentoxifylline
Persantine
Phenylpropanolamine
Prednisone (unless ok'd by your surgeon)
Protamine
Pyrroxate
Ru-Tuss
Saletin
Sinex
Sofarin
Soltice
Sparine
Stelazine
Sulfinpyrazone
Tenuate
Tenuate Dospan
Thorazine
Ticlid
Ticlopidine
Trental
Ursinus
Vibramycin
Vitamin E
Warfarin

Tricyclic Antidepressant Medications to Avoid

Adapin
Amitriptyline
Amoxapine
Anafranil
Asendin
Aventyl
Clomipramine
Desipramine
Doxepin
Elavil
Endep
Etrafon products
Imipramine
Janimine
Limbitrol products
Ludiomil
Maprotiline
Norpramin
Nortriptyline
Pamelor
Pertofrane
Protriptyline

Sinequan
Surmontil
Tofranil
Triavil
Vivactil

Herbal Medications to Avoid

Ginkgo Biloba
Ginseng
St. John's Wort

Going To The Surgery Center

THE OPERATING SUITE
Going to the operating room is not a normal experience for any of us. It is very normal to feel anxious. Your surgeon and all of the professional staff caring for you recognize the natural anxiety with which most patients approach this step in the process of achieving their goals. They believe a description of the surgery experience will be helpful.

Hopefully, your surgery will be performed at a state-of-the-art operating suite. Specialists using modern equipment and techniques will attend to you. The team may include a board-certified anesthesiologist or nurse anesthetist, a trained operating room technician and a registered nurse in charge of the operating room When you arrive at the Surgery Center, you will be escorted to the pre-op area. You will be asked to change into a gown or robe and will be given foot covers. Your surgeon and the anesthesiologist will meet with you before you enter the operating suite. This is the time for final surgical planning; it is also when your surgeon will do basic preparation or draw on your skin as needed. There will be time for last minute questions.

Once you enter the operating room, the staff will do everything they can to make you feel secure. You will be made to feel comfortable on a padded operating table, and the nurse or the anesthesiologist will start an intravenous drip in your arm. At the same time, to ensure your safety, the staff will connect you to monitoring devices. Medicines that will make you drowsy will flow through the tubing into a vein in your arm.

After you are safely and comfortably, your face will be washed with a surgical soap and drapes will be placed around your head to maintain sterility. If your surgery is to be performed under local anesthesia, you may be sedated before the local anesthetic is injected. Lidocaine with epinephrine is most commonly used for the local anesthetic unless you are allergic to it.

For patients having their procedures under local anesthesia, there should be no discomfort after the local anesthesia has been administered. If at any time you are uncomfortable, please let your doctor know. He/She can correct the situation. He/She would like this to be a pleasant experience for you.

When general anesthesia is used, you will be sound asleep and under the care of your anesthesiologist throughout the operation. Once you are settled on the operating table, you will be connected to several monitors and an intravenous catheter. A quick-acting sedative will be given through the intravenous tubing after you have breathed oxygen for a few minutes. Once you fall asleep, your anesthesiologist will usually place an endotracheal tube through your mouth into your windpipe to guarantee that your breathing is safely unimpeded. An anesthetic gas that you will breathe and other medications that will be given through the intravenous catheter will keep you asleep, comfortable and pain free.

The Recovery Area

When your surgery has been completed and your dressings are in place, you will be moved to the recovery room. You will be connected to monitoring equipment constantly. During this period, fully trained recovery personnel will take care of you and remain with you at all times. The registered nurses in the recovery room are specially certified for advanced cardiac life support. The recovery room is likely equipped just like one in a hospital, and that is one of the reasons a Surgery Center is fully accredited.

Your stay in the recovery area will last from 1 to 4 hours, depending on how soon you are ready to leave. Most patients are fully awake within 30-60 minutes after surgery, but may not remember much about their stay in the recovery area.

POST SURGERY ARRANGEMENTS

- AT HOME: You must arrange for someone to bring you to and drive you home from the surgery center. Either a family member, a friend, or a nurse must remain with you the first night after surgery because you will have been sedated.

- HOTEL: Your patient care coordinator can assist with hotel arrangements if desired. Many offices have negotiated reduced rates with several hotels and rooms are available with recliner chairs for your comfort. You may request a room on the ground floor to avoid elevators or stairs.

- RECOVERY CENTER: Occasionally, patients may choose to spend the first night after surgery in the recovery center. This is arranged in advance through your patient care coordinator. However, many patients go home and do fine in this environment.

General Surgical Risks

ABOUT RISKS

You will want to understand fully the risks involved in surgery so that you can make an informed decision. Although complications are infrequent, all surgeries have some degree of risk. Your surgical team will use their expertise and knowledge to avoid complications as much as they are able. If a complication does occur, they will use those same skills to solve the problem quickly. The importance of having a highly qualified medical team and the use of a certified facility cannot be overestimated.

If a complication does arise, your surgeon and the nursing staff will need to cooperate in order to resolve the problem. Most complications involve an extension of the recovery period rather than any permanent effect on your final result.

Normal Symptoms

SWELLING AND BRUISING: Moderate swelling and bruising are completely normal after any surgery. Severe swelling and bruising may indicate bleeding or possible infection.

DISCOMFORT AND PAIN: Mild to moderate discomfort or pain is normal after any surgery. If the pain becomes severe and is not relieved by pain medication, please call your physician. If it is after hours, your surgeon or someone on call can be reached during the evenings and weekends. During evenings and weekends, a physician covering emergency call should be able to be reached through the office telephone number. Make sure this is the case prior to scheduling surgery.

CRUSTING ALONG THE INCISION LINES: Keep incision lines clean and moist with petroleum jelly.

NUMBNESS: Small sensory nerves to the skin surface are occasionally cut when the incision is made or interrupted by undermining of the skin during surgery. The sensation in those areas gradually returns —usually within 2 or 3 months as the nerve endings heal spontaneously.

ITCHING: Itching and occasional small shooting electrical sensations within the skin frequently occur as the nerve endings heal. Ice, skin moisturizers, and massages are frequently helpful. These symptoms are common during the recovery period.

REDNESS OF SCARS: All new scars are red or dark pink. Scars on the face usually fade within 3 to 6 months.

Risks

HEMATOMA: Small collections of blood under the skin are usually allowed to absorb spontaneously. Larger hematomas may require aspiration or surgical drainage to achieve the best result.

INFLAMMATION AND INFECTION: An infection may require antibiotic medication. Development of an abscess usually requires drainage. Occasionally, deep sutures may become infected and need to be removed through a small incision.

THICK, WIDE OR DEPRESSED SCARS: Abnormal scars may occur even though your surgeon has used the most modern plastic surgery techniques. Injection of steroids in to the scars, placement of silicone gel on the scars or further surgery to correct the scars may be necessary. Some areas on the body scar more than others, and some people scar more than others. The nose heals very well and usually faster than other areas of the body.

WOUND SEPARATION OR DELAYED HEALING: Any incision, during the healing phase, may separate or heal unusually slow for a number of reasons. These include inflammation, infection, wound tension, decreased circulation, smoking or excess external pressure. If delayed healing occurs, the final outcome is usually not significantly affected, but revision of the scar may be beneficial in rare cases.

SENSITIVITY OR ALLERGY TO DRESSINGS OR TAPE: Occasionally, allergic or sensitivity reactions may occur from soaps, ointments, tape or sutures used during or after surgery. Such problems are unusual and are usually mild and easily treated. In extremely rare circumstances, allergic reactions may need more aggressive treatment.

INCREASED RISKS FOR SMOKERS: Smokers have a greater chance of skin loss and poor healing because of decreased skin circulation. (See Preparing for Surgery)

INJURY TO DEEPER STRUCTURES: Blood vessels, nerves and muscles may be injured during surgery. The incidence of such injuries is extremely rare.

Rarer Complications

If they are severe, any of the problems mentioned above under the Risks section may significantly delay healing or necessitate further surgical procedures.

Medical complications such as pulmonary embolism, severe allergic reactions to medications, cardiac arrhythmias, heart attack and hyperthermia are rare, but serious and life-threatening problems. Having a board-certified anesthesiologist or certified registered nurse anesthetist present at your surgery reduces these risks as much as possible. (Failure to disclose all pertinent medical data before surgery may cause serious problems for you and for the medical team during surgery.)

Be honest and forthcoming about all your medical history prior to surgery.

Unsatisfactory Result & Need For Revisional Surgery

All facial plastic surgery treatments and operations are performed to improve a condition, a problem or appearance. While the procedures are performed with a very high probability of success, disappointments occur and results are not always acceptable to patients or the surgeon. Secondary procedures or treatments may be indicated. Rarely, problems may occur that are permanent.

POOR RESULTS: To some extent, the human body and the way it heals can be unpredictable. Asymmetry, unhappiness with the result or poor healing may occur. Minimal differences are usually acceptable. Larger differences usually benefit from revisional surgery.

Specific Surgical Risks
Rhinoplasty (Nose Reshaping)

NEED FOR FURTHER SURGERY: If asymmetry or an undesired contour is present after surgery, an additional small surgical procedure can be performed to improve the appearance.

SWELLING: It typically takes 10-12 months for <u>ALL</u> swelling to disappear and for your final result to be achieved.

SCARRING: Internal scarring or adhesions may occur, but are unlikely complications.

DECREASED SENSATION: Reduced sensation or numbness generally occurs (usually in the nasal tip) following rhinoplasty. The sensation gradually returns over nine months, although sometimes not completely.

NASAL OBSTRUCTION: Possible healing problems may occur which may result in the airways remaining blocked or obstructed causing difficulty in breathing. Obstruction from swelling is expected during the early recovery period.

INJURY TO ADJACENT STRUCTURES AND NASAL FUNCTION: Injury to nerves, tear ducts, muscles and sense of smell are very rare, but can potentially occur.

PERFORATED NASAL SEPTUM: A permanent hole (perforation) developing through the septum (divider between the two sides of the nose) is a remote possibility following nasal surgery. Most small perforations have no symptoms. In rare cases, further surgical correction may be indicated. Very rarely, the septal perforation cannot be corrected.

TIP SWELLING: There may be persistent swelling in the nose, especially around the tip, that may be temporary, last several months or years, or may be permanent.

VOICE CHANGE: The patient may notice changes in the sound of their voice (uncommon). If the surgery is done to correct obstruction of the nose, the voice may be less "nasal", clearer, or more resonant after healing from surgery.

SADDLE DEFORMITY: Rarely, following extensive septal surgery, the nasal profile above the nasal tip can become depressed because of partial loss of cartilage support. Should this occur, secondary corrective surgery may be recommended.

NOSTRIL ASYMMETRY: A deviated nasal septum frequently causes one nostril to look larger than the other because the deviation pushes the columella (the divider between the two nostrils) to one side. Even though the septal correction may improve breathing, all of the nostril asymmetry may not disappear. This is typical even under the best circumstances.

ALTERNATIVES: Not having the surgery will eliminate the risks. After all, it is your decision whether or not to have surgery.

Applicable Health Factors
SPECIAL INFORMATION FOR PATIENTS WITH
MITRAL VALVE PROLAPSE

The heart is a hollow, muscular organ with four chambers. The heart valves are like one-way doors. They open to let blood through and close to keep blood from flowing backwards. Sometimes heart valves open and close in different ways. Such is the case of mitral valve prolapse.

Mitral valve prolapse (MVP) is a minor heart condition. Very little treatment (if any) is needed, but there are precautions and symptoms you should know. MVP does not put you at higher risk of a heart attack. Many people with MVP do, however, have a greater chance of getting infective or bacterial endocarditis. This is an infection of the heart valves or inner heart lining that can cause scarring or damage to the valves.

ANTIBIOTICS
For these reasons, you may consider taking an antibiotic before you have dental work, surgery, or procedures that cause trauma to body tissues such as bladder or colon examinations. It is important that you take the pre-operative antibiotics as your physician prescribes them.

Other Risks And Information

We have not discussed every possible problem that may occur, and you cannot assume that a problem will not occur simply because it is not discussed here.

Please acknowledge to yourself that the risks and complications of the surgery you are considering have been explained and discussed with you in detail by your surgeon and by the nursing staff. You should have been given the opportunity to ask questions and any concerns you had about your surgery have been explained to you.

On the following pages, a sample consent is provided that may be similar to the one used by your surgeon. This should not be considered all-inclusive. Hopefully you find it helpful to review prior to your surgery or decision to proceed with surgery.

Sample Rhinoplasty Consent Form

Consent For Surgery

I, (patient), desire (surgeon), and such assistants as may be assigned by him/her to perform the elective procedure(s) of

COSMETIC RHINOPLASTY (Surgery to improve the appearance of my nose)

The nature and purpose of the operation(s), possible alternative methods of treatment, including no treatment/surgery, risks and possible complications have been fully explained to me by my surgeon during my preoperative consultation. I understand that this operation is not an emergency, nor is it medically necessary to improve or protect my physical health. I have been advised that all surgery involves general risks, including but not limited to bleeding, infection, nerve or tissue damage and, rarely, cardiac arrest, death, or other serious bodily injury. I acknowledge that no guarantees or assurances have been made as to the results that may be obtained.

I understand that anesthesia will be given and that it, too, carries risks. I consent to the administration of anesthesia by either my surgeon or a qualified anesthesiologist and to the use of such anesthetics, as he/she may deem advisable.

It has been explained to me that during the course of the operation, unforeseen conditions may be revealed that necessitate an extension of the original procedure, and I hereby authorize my doctor and/or such assistants as may be selected by him/her to perform such procedures as are necessary and desirable, including but not limited to the services of pathologists, radiologists, or a laboratory. The authority granted in this paragraph shall extend to remedying conditions that are not known to my doctor at the time the operation commences.

I understand that if computer generated photographs were used in my planning that it was used merely for the purpose of illustration and discussion. I certify my understanding that there is not a warranty, expressed or implied as to my final appearance by the use of such electronically altered images.

I hereby authorize my surgeon or his/her assistants to take photographs of me before, during or after my operation. I permit such photographs to be used for medical education, general information, knowledge or research. I relinquish all title and interest in these photographs to my surgeon. Photos will not be used for publication or general display without a separate consent form for this purpose.

I agree to keep my doctor informed of any change in my permanent address so that he/she can inform me of any important new findings relating to my surgery. I further agree to cooperate with him/her in my aftercare until I am discharged from his/her care.

In signing this consent, I hereby certify that I understand the risks, benefits, and alternatives to my procedure(s) and that I have discussed them with my surgeon.

Please do not give your permission or sign this consent form if you have any questions regarding your procedure(s). Please advise a staff member of these questions or concerns so that arrangements can be made for your surgeon to discuss them with you.

Signature: _____
Date: _____

Witness: _____
Relationship: _____

Medications

GENERAL INFORMATION
The doctor and the nursing staff may give you prescriptions for your comfort and care. It is important that you use the medications as directed unless you experience abnormal symptoms that might be related to medication usage.

You will likely be given prescriptions for medications, which may be used during the recovery period. You may also be given antibiotic capsules or a prescription for antibiotics depending on the procedure you are undergoing. Many pain medications can cause nausea, so the goal with this pain control regimen is to achieve adequate pain control with little risk of nausea.

Using the medications as instructed will help reduce the risk of nausea, while achieving maximum pain control.

Symptoms such as itching, development of a rash, wheezing, and tightness in the throat may be due to an allergy. Should these occur, discontinue all medications and call the surgeon's office for instructions. If it is after normal office hours, your surgeon or someone on call can often be reached during evenings and weekends via the office phone number.

During evenings and weekends, a physician covering emergency calls can always be reached through the office telephone number. Make sure this is the case prior to surgery.

Instructions

PAIN: Many postoperative pain medications are strong narcotics and can cause nausea, particularly at larger doses. The general dosage of many prescription pain medications 1-2 tablets every four hours, but it may be preferable to take one half tablet every hour or so with food. This lessens the strength of each dose, and the potential nauseating effect, while still providing the same overall dosage in a four-hour time span. This medication must be taken with food to reduce the risk of nausea. An individual container of applesauce, yogurt, pudding or other soft food works well to lessen the impact on the stomach and drinking fluids is also beneficial.

If you are having only a little discomfort after surgery, you can try acetaminophen instead of the narcotic medications for additional pain control. Do not use acetaminophen during the same time span as the other because both medications may contain acetaminophen.

If you become nauseated: Nausea immediately following surgery may be due to the anesthetic administered. This may start in the recovery room and improves with time. Nausea that develops later on is most often due to the pain medications, particularly the narcotics. If you are experiencing nausea, try to avoid using the narcotic because this may be the most likely cause of the nausea. Persistent discomfort with nausea causing vomiting may necessitate a call to you physician.

MEDICATIONS

POST OP ANTIBIOTICS: Antibiotics may reduce the likelihood of a postoperative infection. Use antibiotics <u>only as directed</u>. Please note that many antibiotics can affect the function of birth control pills and any antibiotic can cause upset stomach or diarrhea or even yeast infections. If this occurs, do not take the next dose and call your surgeon's office to ask about your next option. Most symptoms resolve soon after stopping the antibiotic.

Postoperative Care Outpatient Surgery Your First 48 Hours

IMPORTANT: If at any time you have excessive pain, nausea and vomiting, temperature of more than 101 degrees, over sedation, or any other concerns, please call your surgeon. If it is after normal office hours, your surgeon can often be reached during the evenings and weekends at home. During weekends and evenings, a physician covering emergency calls can always be reached through the office telephone number.

YOUR FIRST 24 HOURS: If you are going home, a family member or friend must drive you because you have been sedated. Someone must stay overnight with you.

MEDICATIONS: Take the prescribed medication as directed and resume your normal medications except for products containing aspirin, ibuprofen, Vitamin E, fish oils or medicinal herbs.

DRESSINGS: Keep your dressings as clean and dry as possible. Do not remove them unless instructed to do so.

DIET: You are encouraged to eat and drink following surgery. This will lessen the chances of stomach irritation and nausea from your pain pills. You may wish to have a supply of applesauce, yogurt, pudding, or other soft foods that are available in individual containers for your convenience.

ACTIVITY: Take it easy and pamper yourself. Try to avoid any straining. You may go to the bathroom, sit and watch TV, etc., but no matter how good you feel, do not clean the house, rearrange the attic, etc. Your surgeon does not want you to bleed and cause any more swelling and bruising than is unavoidable.

POSITION: Elevating your head after surgery will lessen the swelling. It is therefore helpful to sleep in a recliner or on your back in bed with several pillows under your head and back. A cushion can be placed under the mattress to further raise the head of the bed. Continue sleeping with your head elevated for several days to lessen swelling.

SWELLING: Every operation, no matter how minor, is accompanied by swelling of the surrounding tissues. The amount varies from person to person and is generally greater on the second day after surgery. There is typically more in the face because of the looseness of the tissues and because even a small amount makes the features appear distorted. The swelling itself is not serious and is not an indication that something is going wrong with your recovery process.

BRUISING: Bruising will generally clear by 10 to 14 days after surgery. Everyone heals differently. The amount of bruising and swelling varies from patient to patient.

SMOKING: Smoking reduces capillary flow in your skin. Your surgeon will likely advise you not to smoke at all during the first 2 weeks after surgery.

ALCOHOL: Alcohol dilates the blood vessels and could increase postoperative bleeding. Do not drink alcohol until you have stopped taking the prescription pain pills, as the combination of pain pills and alcohol can be dangerous.

DRIVING: Do not drive for at least 2 days after general anesthesia or intravenous sedation or while taking prescription pain pills.

POST OPERATIVE APPOINTMENTS: It is very important that you follow the schedule of appointments established after surgery.

Specific Post Operative Instructions Rhinoplasty (Nose Reshaping)

ICE MASK: You may be given a gelatin mask at the surgery facility, which will be used to cool your eyes. Place this in ice water for 1 to 2 minutes to chill it, and then drape it across your eyes for 10 minutes or so to help reduce swelling and bruising. Repeat this procedure during the first 24 hours after surgery except while sleeping. Use of the cold mask beyond 24 hours is usually ineffective but may provide comfort.

DRESSINGS: At the conclusion of the procedure, a splint may be placed on the nose and dressings may be inserted in to both nostrils. If they are used, the intranasal dressings may be removed the following morning and the splint and sutures will be removed after 4 to 6 days. You will be able to breathe through your nose somewhat even with the dressings in place.

WOUND CARE: Change the gauze drip pad under your nose as needed. A moderate amount of mucous and bloody drainage is expected the first 24 hours after surgery. It is normal to need to change the nasal drip pad every hour or so.

Mouth breathing due to postoperative intranasal swelling can cause dryness. Drinking plenty of fluids and using a humidifier in your bedroom if needed will improve the dryness.

Do not blow your nose for up to 2 weeks. Secretions may be sniffed. Frequent use of saline nasal spray will moisturize your nose and it may be used as often as desired. The nasal spray can be used 6-8 times per day during the first two weeks after surgery.

You may swab the suture lines just inside your nostrils with Q-tips and water, or hydrogen peroxide 3 times daily. After each cleansing, apply a pea-sized amount of petroleum jelly to the inside of the nostrils. If your surgeon used absorbable sutures inside the nose, you may notice tan-colored stitches working loose during these cleansings. This is of no concern. The saline nasal spray and petroleum jelly use may be continued for several months as needed to prevent dryness inside the nose. The same wound care is used for any external suture lines around the nostrils if any are present.

HAIR CARE: You may wash your hair after surgery and the splint can get wet. Simply blot the splint dry when you complete your shower. Ask your individual surgeon, but this is generally the case.

As You Heal

FAMILY & FRIENDS
Support from family and friends is very helpful, but because they may not understand what constitutes a normal postoperative course, their comments may unintentionally create emotional turmoil for you. Your surgeon will tell you honestly how you are doing and what he or she expects your result to be. Please trust in the knowledge and experience of your surgeon when he or she discusses your progress with you.

Although plastic surgery has certainly "come out of the closet" in the past decade, your friends may still be reluctant to bring up and discuss what they believe is a private matter. Patients occasionally feel upset that "no one noticed" or "said anything". If you feel comfortable discussing your surgical experience, do so openly. When people ask how you are, respond by saying, "I feel wonderful. I just had cosmetic surgery and I'm recovering." This lets people know that they may talk freely with you. Often when patients are open, they find that their friends and acquaintances are very interested in discussing the subject.

DEPRESSION
Quite frequently patients may experience a brief period of let-down or depression after cosmetic surgery. Some may subconsciously have expected to feel and look better instantly, even though they rationally understand that this will not be the case. Patients commonly question their decision to have surgery during the first few days after surgery. As the healing occurs, these thoughts usually disappear quickly. If you feel depressed, understanding that this is a natural phase of the healing process may help you to cope with this emotional state.

HEALING
Everyone has the capacity to heal him or herself to one degree or another. Clearly, this ability is variable and depends upon a number of factors such as

your genetic background, your overall state of health and lifestyle (exercise, diet, smoking, drinking, etc.). Your surgeon can facilitate (but not accelerate) the healing process. Your cooperation and close attention is extremely important and in your best interest.

Specific As You Heal Information Rhinoplasty (Nose Reshaping)

NUMBNESS AND SWELLING: You may experience some degree of numbness of the tip of your nose for up to nine months or longer. You may have some swelling for up to 12 months, and the incision site inside the nose may remain swollen or feel firm for many months after surgery.

INCREASED SWELLING: Intermittent increases in swelling will occur for the first few weeks to months after surgery. This is usually more noticeable early in the morning.

DRIPPING: You may want to carry some tissues with you for a number of weeks after surgery, since your nose may "drip". This is because the inside of your nose may have some temporary numbness and is inefficient and "over effective" at moisturizing the inside of your nose. This usually improves and resolves throughout the healing process.

ACTIVITIES/WORK: Many people feel quite "normal" within 5-10 days. If your work keeps you sedentary, you may return when you are able. Heavy exercise or straining can cause bleeding or swelling during the first 2-3 weeks.

Longer Term Postoperative Instructions

ACTIVITY/SPORTS: Since you have undergone a major surgical operation, you will have restrictions in your activities post-operatively. Avoid exercise regimens and any lifting of more than 10 lbs. (the weight of a gallon of fluid) or straining for 2 weeks after surgery. It is acceptable to do some light walking 3 days after surgery. Jogging and non-contact exercise should not be resumed until 3 weeks post-operatively and strenuous sports require 4 weeks of healing before being safely resumed. The same general restrictions apply to sexual activities.

RETIN-A: Retin-A or alpha-hydroxy acid skin care may be resumed 2 weeks after surgery.

MAKE-UP: Do not apply make-up over the incisions for several days after the sutures are removed, and never apply it over an area of crusting. Make-up can, however, be brought up close to the line of the incision. Water-based make-up may be used over the incision after the sutures are removed and there has been no crusting for 2 days.

SUN EXPOSURE: Exposure to the sun (including sun tanning salons) in the first 3 weeks after surgery may result in prolonged facial swelling and injury to the skin. Thereafter, you should always protect your skin with a strong sunscreen (SPF 15 or greater) to decrease the aging effects of pigmentation change caused by the sun.

FATIGUE: You may be up and around the day after surgery, but it is natural for some fatigue to persist for 2 to 3 days due to the normal effects of the anesthesia and the surgical procedure. This will quickly resolve.

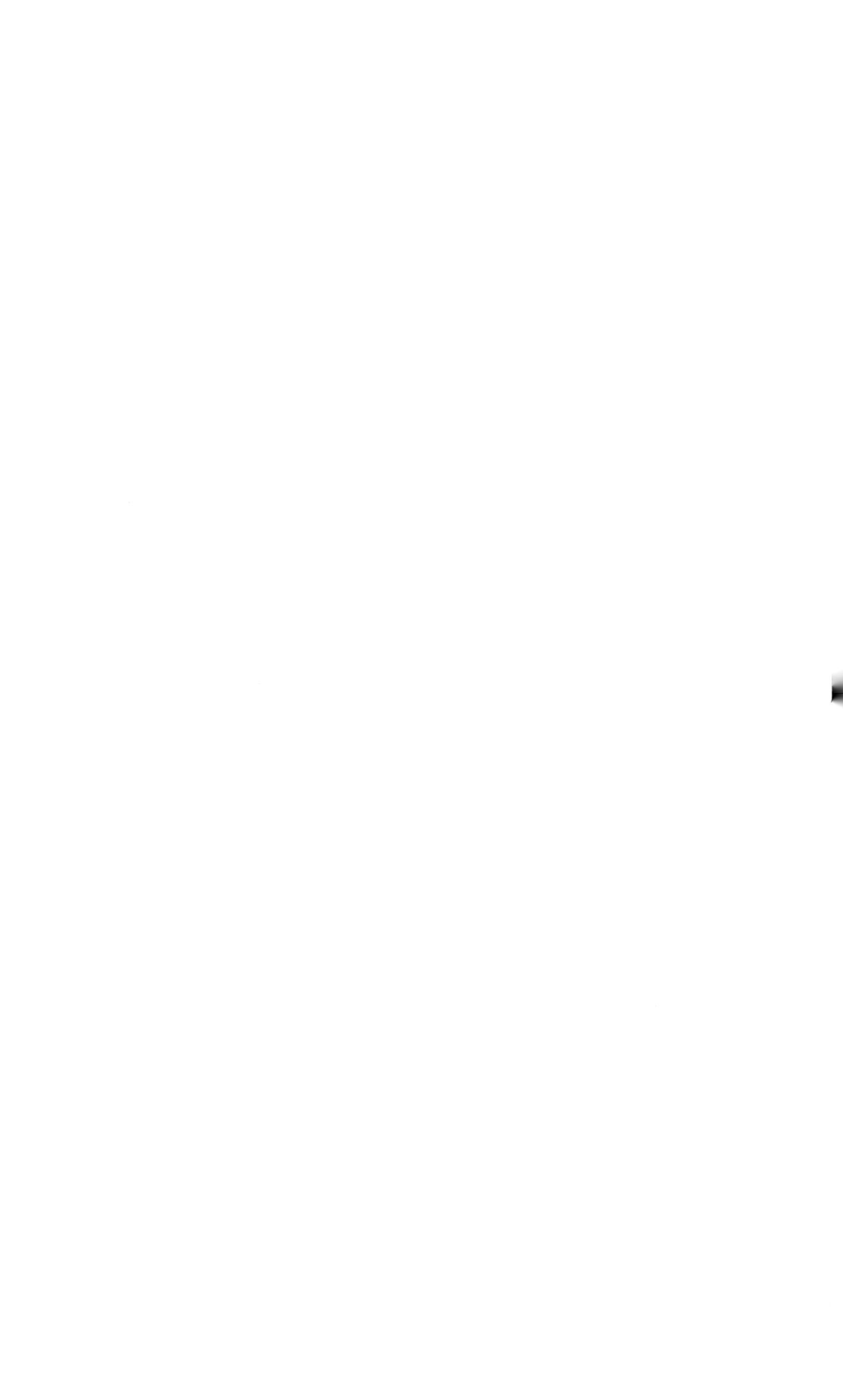

Finally

Relax! Pamper yourself a little. A positive mental outlook can help speed healing and foster feelings of well-being.

Congratulations for taking this significant step toward improved health and well-being. Your surgeon, no doubt, greatly appreciates the confidence you have shown in him/her and you can be assured of their best effort to achieve the most satisfactory result possible for your particular situation.

www.ingramcontent.com/pod-product-compliance
Lightning Source LLC
Chambersburg PA
CBHW061517180526
45171CB00001B/218